Abdel Bacite Zarouali
Hicham Elmsellem
Zahra Ba-aqqa

Investigation of Decubitus Complications in the Intensive Care Unit

Abdel Bacite Zarouali
Hicham Elmsellem
Zahra Ba-aqqa

Investigation of Decubitus Complications in the Intensive Care Unit

ScienciaScripts

Imprint
Any brand names and product names mentioned in this book are subject to trademark, brand or patent protection and are trademarks or registered trademarks of their respective holders. The use of brand names, product names, common names, trade names, product descriptions etc. even without a particular marking in this work is in no way to be construed to mean that such names may be regarded as unrestricted in respect of trademark and brand protection legislation and could thus be used by anyone.

Cover image: www.ingimage.com

This book is a translation from the original published under ISBN 978-620-6-71606-8.

Publisher:
Sciencia Scripts
is a trademark of
Dodo Books Indian Ocean Ltd. and OmniScriptum S.R.L publishing group

120 High Road, East Finchley, London, N2 9ED, United Kingdom
Str. Armeneasca 28/1, office 1, Chisinau MD-2012, Republic of Moldova, Europe
Printed at: see last page
ISBN: 978-620-7-84822-5

DESCRIPTIVE STUDY ON THE MANAGEMENT OF DECUBITUS COMPLICATIONS IN INTENSIVE CARE UNITS

"Decubitus complications in the intensive care unit" is a book which focuses on a descriptive study of the management of decubitus complications in the intensive care unit. The book addresses the various aspects of this problem, starting with an introduction that presents the context of the study, its objectives, the methodology used and the study's limitations.

The second chapter looks at decubitus complications in the ICU, defining these complications, identifying the associated risk factors and examining the impact they can have on patients. Prevention strategies are also discussed in this chapter.

The third chapter focuses on the management of decubitus complications, describing the initial assessment of the patient, possible medical treatments, surgical interventions that may be necessary, and the nursing care and rehabilitation that must be put in place. Clinical cases are also studied to illustrate the different situations encountered.

The following chapters explore the results of the study, analysing the characteristics of the patients included, the prevalence of decubitus complications, the factors associated with these complications and the effectiveness of the treatments used. A discussion is then held to interpret these results, compare them with other studies, identify the limitations of the study and proposefuture prospects. Finally, a conclusion summarises the results, highlights the clinical implications and makes recommendations.

Key words : *Pressure sores; Decubitus; Skin complications; Resuscitation; Lying position; Bedridden; Change of position.*

1. INTRODUCTION

1.1 Background to the study

Decubitus complications are common health problems in intensive care patients. These complications arise from the patient's prolonged position in a bed or on a hard surface, which causes excessive pressure on certain parts of the body. The areas most affected are generally the heels, buttocks, elbows and back.The management of decubitus complications is a major challenge for healthcare professionals in intensive care. These complications can lead to pain, infection, pressure ulcers and even amputation in the most serious cases. They also prolong the length of stay in intensive care and increase healthcare costs. It is therefore essential to understand the risk factors, consequences and best practices for prevention and treatment of decubitus complications. The aim of this descriptive study is to examine the management of decubitus complications in the intensive care unit, focusing on initial patient assessment, medical treatment, surgical interventions, nursing care and rehabilitation. The study will be conducted in a university hospital, where intensive care patients will be included in the study. Data will be collected from patients' medical records, using a rigorous methodology to ensure the reliability of the results. The main aim of this study is to evaluate the effectiveness of different approaches to the management of decubitus complications in intensive care. The specific objectives are as follows:

1. To examine the characteristics of the patients included in the study, such as age, sex, medical history and length of stay in intensive care.
2. To determine the prevalence of decubitus complications in intensive care patients.
3. Identify the factors associated with the development of decubitus complications, such as immobility, malnutrition, the presence of co-morbidities and the use of certain medications.
4. To assess the effectiveness of medical treatments used to prevent and treat decubitus complications.
5. To analyse the results of surgical interventions carried out to treat decubitus complications.
6. To examine the impact of nursing care and rehabilitation on the prevention and treatment of decubitus complications.

The results of this study will provide valuable information on the management of decubitus complications in the ICU. These results can be used to improve clinical practice, develop more effective prevention and treatment protocols, and improve clinical outcomes for intensive care patients.

It should be noted that this study has certain limitations. Firstly, it will be conducted in a single hospital centre, which may limit the generalisability of the results. In addition, the collection of data from medical records may lead to documentation errors. Despite these limitations, this study will provide valuable information on the management of decubitus complications in the ICU, which can be used to improve patient care.

1.1 Aims of the study

The aim of this descriptive study was to analyse the management of decubitus complications in the intensive care unit. Decubitus complications are health problems that occur in patients confined to bed for long periods, particularly in intensive care units. These complications can have serious consequences for patients' health, increasing their morbidity and mortality.

The aim of the study was to examine the different management strategies for decubitus complications implemented in the intensive care unit, focusing on the initial assessment of the patient, medical treatment, surgical interventions, and nursing care and rehabilitation. More specifically, the objectives of this study are as follows:

1.1.1 Evaluate the effectiveness of management strategies currently in use

The aim of the study is to evaluate the effectiveness of the different management strategies for decubitus complications implemented in the intensive care unit. This includes evaluation of the effectiveness of treatments medical treatment used, the surgical procedures performed, and the nursing care and rehabilitation provided to patients. The aim is to determine whether these management strategies reduce the prevalence of decubitus complications and improve patients' clinical outcomes.

1.1.2 Identifying factors associated with decubitus complications

Another aim of this study is to identify the factors associated with the development of decubitus complications in intensive care patients. This includes analysis of risk factors such as age, gender, general health, length of bed rest and other factors specific to the ICU. Identifying these factors will provide a better understanding of the causes of decubitus complications and enable targeted preventive measures to be put in place.

1.1.3 Propose recommendations to improve the management of decubitus complications

Finally, this study aims to formulate recommendations for improving the management of decubitus complications in the intensive care unit. These recommendations will be based on the results of the study and a review of the existing literature. The aim is to identify best practice in the prevention, assessment and treatment of decubitus complications, in order to improve patients' clinical outcomes and reduce their morbidity and mortality.

In summary, this descriptive study of the management of decubitus complications in the intensive care unit aims to assess the effectiveness of the strategies currently used, to identify the factors associated with these complications, and to formulate recommendations for improving patient management. The results of this study could help to improve clinical practice and reduce decubitus complications in intensive care patients.

1.2 Methodology

In this section, we describe the methodology used to conduct our descriptive study on the management of decubitus complications in the intensive care unit. We will explain the different stages of our study, including patient selection, data collection and statistical analysis.

1.2.1 Study population

Our study was conducted in an intensive care unit of a university hospital. The study population included all patients admitted to the intensive care unit over a six-month period. The inclusion criteria were as follows: patients aged 18 and over, requiring intensive care admission and presenting with decubitus complications.

1.2.2 Data collection

Data were collected from patients' medical records. Variables collected included patient demographics (age, gender), medical history, co-morbidities, length of stay in intensive care, decubitus complications encountered, treatments administered and clinical outcomes.

1.2.3 Data analysis

The data collected was analysed using SPSS (Statistical Package for the Social Sciences) statistical software. Quantitative variables were expressed as mean ± standard deviation, while qualitative variables were expressed as a percentage.

Comparisons between groups were made using the Student's t test for continuous variables and the chi-square test for categorical variables. A p-value of less than 0.05 was considered statistically significant.

1.2.4 Research ethics

This study was conducted in accordance with the ethical principles of the Declaration of Helsinki. The study was approved by our institution's ethics committee. All patients' personal details were anonymised and the data were treated as confidential.

1.2.5 Limitations of the study

Our study has certain limitations. Firstly, due to its descriptive nature, it cannot establish a cause and effect relationship between decubitus complications and the risk factors identified. Secondly, our study was conducted in a single intensive care unit, which limits the generalisability of the results to other settings. Finally, data collection from medical records may result in documentation errors or missing data. Despite these limitations, our study provides valuable information on the management of decubitus complications in the intensive care unit. The results obtained could help to improve clinical practice and reduce the morbidity associated with these complications. In conclusion, our descriptive study of the management of decubitus complications in the intensive care unit used a rigorous methodology to collect and analyse the data. The results of this study will be presented in Chapter 5 and discussed in Chapter 6 of this book.

1.3 Limitations of the study

The study we carried out on the management of decubitus complications in the intensive care unit has certain limitations which it is important to take into account when interpreting the results.

1.3.1 Sample size

One of the main limitations of our study is the size of the sample. Due to time and resource constraints, we were able to include a limited number of patients in our study. Consequently, the results obtained may not be generalisable to the entire population of intensive care patients. Subsequent studies with larger samples are therefore necessary to confirm our results.

1.3.2 Selection bias

Another potential bias in our study is selection bias. The patients included in our study were selected non-randomly, which may introduce bias into the results.

For example, if patients with more severe decubitus complications were excluded from the study, this could underestimate the prevalence of these complications. of these complications. It is therefore important to take this bias into account when interpreting the results.

1.3.3 Measurement bias

Another aspect to consider is measurement bias. Decubitus complications were assessed by medical and nursing staff in the intensive care unit, which may introduce bias in the assessment of complications. Although care was taken to train staff in the use of standardised criteria to assess decubitus complications, it is possible that variations in assessment may have occurred. This may influence the results of the study and should therefore be taken into account when interpreting the results.

1.3.4 Retrospective of the study

Our study is retrospective in nature, which means that we analysed patients' medical records to collect the data. This approach may lead to limitations, such as missing or incomplete data. In addition, some events may not have been correctly recorded in the medical records, which may affect the accuracy of the results. It is therefore important to take these limitations into account when interpreting the results.

1.3.5 Confounding factors

Finally, it is important to note that our study did not take into account all potential confounding factors. There are many factors that can influence the development of decubitus complications, such as age, general health, length of stay in intensive care, etc. Although we adjusted our analyses for some of these factors, it is possible that other unmeasured factors may have influenced the development of decubitus complications. Although we have adjusted our analyses for some of these factors, it is possible that other unmeasured factors may have influenced the results. It is therefore important to take this limitation into account when interpreting the results. Despite these limitations, our study provides valuable information on the management of decubitus complications in the intensive care unit. These results may serve as a basis for future research and contribute to improving clinical practice in this area.

2. DECUBITUS COMPLICATIONS IN INTENSIVE CARE

2.1 Definition of decubitus complications

Decubitus complications, also known as bedsores, are skin lesions that develop in patients who are bedridden or immobilised for long periods. They occur mainly in pressure areas such as the heels, buttocks, elbows and back. Decubitus complications are a major concern in intensive care, as they can lead to pain, infection and delays in patient recovery.

Decubitus complications are classified into several stages, ranging from stage 1 to stage 4, depending on their severity. In stage 1, the skin is red and does not go away when the pressure is released. In stage 2, the skin is damaged and has a superficial wound. In stage 3, the wound extends deeper, reaching the subcutaneous tissue. In stage 4, the wound is deep and exposes muscles, tendons and bones.

Decubitus complications are mainly caused by prolonged pressure on the skin, which compresses the blood vessels and limits the supply of oxygen and nutrients to the tissues. This leads to tissue necrosis and the formation of bedsores. Other risk factors can also contribute to the development of decubitus complications, such as excessive humidity, friction, malnutrition, dehydration, incontinence and poor hygiene.

The consequences of decubitus complications can be serious, leading to further medical complications. Patients with pressure sores can suffer from severe pain, infection, sepsis, delayed healing, reduced quality of life and even death. In addition, decubitus complications can prolong the length of stay of patients in intensive care, increasing the cost of care and the workload of medical staff.

Prevention of decubitus complications is essential to reduce the incidence of these skin lesions in intensive care patients. Preventive measures must be put in place as soon as the patient is admitted, with regular assessment of the patient's skin condition. risk of developing pressure sores and by implementing appropriate prevention strategies. These strategies include regular patient rotation, the use of special mattresses and cushions to reduce pressure, maintaining good skin hygiene, managing humidity and incontinence, and optimising patient nutrition and hydration. It is also important to make medical and nursing staff aware of the importance of preventing decubitus complications. Adequate training in preventive measures and early recognition of the signs of pressure sores is essential to ensure optimal care for intensive care patients. In addition, interdisciplinary collaboration between doctors, nurses, physiotherapists and nutritionists is needed to put in place a comprehensive, individualised prevention plan for each patient.

In conclusion, decubitus complications are serious skin lesions that can occur in intensive care patients. They are caused by prolonged pressure on the skin and can lead to pain, infection and delayed healing. Preventing decubitus complications is crucial, and requires preventive measures to be put in place as soon as the patient is admitted. Awareness-raising among medical and nursing staff and interdisciplinary collaboration are essential to ensure optimal patient management and reduce the incidence of decubitus complications in the intensive care unit.

2.2 Risk factors

Decubitus complications in intensive care can occur in the most vulnerable patients, particularly those who are bedridden for long periods. Several risk factors can contribute to the development of these complications. It is essential to identify them in order to implement appropriate preventive measures and reduce the harmful consequences for patients.

2.2.1 Prolonged immobility

Prolonged immobility is one of the main risk factors for decubitus complications in intensive care. When patients remain bedridden for long periods, the pressure exerted on the areas in contact with the bed or mattress can lead to a reduction in blood circulation and a build-up of pressure. on the skin. This can lead to the formation of bedsores, which are serious skin lesions.

2.2.2 Malnutrition

Malnutrition is another major risk factor for decubitus complications in intensive care. Patients who do not receive adequate nutrition may experience reduced skin resistance and impaired wound healing. A balanced, nutrient-rich diet is essential to maintain skin integrity and prevent decubitus complications.

2.2.3 Incontinence

Urinary or faecal incontinence can considerably increase the risk of decubitus complications in intensive care. Excessive moisture on the skin can lead to maceration and fragility of the skin, making patients more vulnerable to skin lesions. It is therefore essential to maintain adequate hygiene and take steps to prevent incontinence in intensive care patients.

2.2.4 Advanced age

The elderly are more likely to develop decubitus complications in intensive care due to the fragility of their skin and their reduced capacity for cell regeneration. In addition, the elderly may have other underlying health problems that increase their vulnerability to skin lesions. Particular attention must therefore be paid to preventing decubitus complications in elderly patients.

2.2.5 Chronic diseases

Patients with chronic illnesses, such as diabetes, renal failure or cardiovascular disease, are more likely to develop decubitus complications in intensive care. These diseases can affect blood circulation, wound healing and skin resistance, increasing the risk of skin lesions. Specific management must be put in place for these patients to prevent decubitus complications.

2.2.6 Obesity

Obesity is a major risk factor for decubitus complications in intensive care. Obese patients have increased pressure on areas in contact with the bed or mattress, which can lead to reduced blood circulation and pressure build-up on the skin. Obesity can also make it more difficult to manage skin lesions and prevent complications.

2.2.7 Smoking

Smoking is an additional risk factor for decubitus complications in intensive care. Smoking impairs blood circulation and wound healing, which can increase the risk of skin lesions in intensive care patients. It is therefore recommended that patients be encouraged to stop smoking before and during their stay in intensive care.

2.2.8 Medicines

Certain drugs can increase the risk of decubitus complications in intensive care. For example, corticosteroids can weaken the skin and reduce resistance to skin lesions. Similarly, certain drugs used to treat certain chronic diseases can affect blood circulation and wound healing. It is important to take these factors into account when managing patients in intensive care.

2.2.9 Other factors

Other risk factors may also contribute to the development of decubitus complications in intensive care, such as the presence of pre-existing wounds or scars, poor hygiene, poor patient positioning on the bed, poor mattress support, etc. It is essential to take all these factors into account when assessing the risk of decubitus complications in intensive care patients. It is essential to take all these factors into account when assessing the risk of decubitus complications in intensive care patients.

In conclusion, several risk factors may contribute to the development of decubitus complications in intensive care. It is essential to identify these risk factors in order to implement appropriate preventive measures and reduce the adverse consequences for patients. A multidisciplinary approach and individualised management are needed to effectively prevent decubitus complications in the ICU.

2.3 Consequences of decubitus complications

Decubitus complications in intensive care can have serious consequences for patients' health. These complications can lead to a deterioration in the patient's general condition, prolong the length of their stay in intensive care and increase the risk of subsequent complications. In this section, we will examine the various consequences of decubitus complications and their impact on the management of intensive care patients.

2.3.1 Infections

One of the most frequent consequences of decubitus complications in intensive care is infection. Decubitus wounds can become entry points for bacteria, which can lead to local or systemic infection. Infections associated with decubitus wounds can be difficult to treat due to the presence of bacteria that are multi-resistant to antibiotics. In addition, these infections can prolong the length of stay in intensive care and increase the risk of serious complications, such as septicaemia.

2.3.2 Pain and discomfort

Decubitus complications can cause severe pain and discomfort in intensive care patients. Decubitus wounds can be extremely painful, which can make pain management difficult for these patients. In addition, intensive care patients are often immobilised and bedridden, which can lead to muscle and joint pain. Pain and discomfort can have a negative impact on patients' quality of life and their ability to participate in rehabilitation.

2.3.3 Delayed healing

Decubitus wounds in intensive care tend to heal more slowly than other types of wound. This may be due to a number of factors, such as the presence of infections, poor circulation and malnutrition. Delayed healing can prolong the length of stay in intensive care and increase the risk of further complications. It is therefore essential to implement appropriate prevention and treatment measures to promote the healing of decubitus wounds.

2.3.4 Deterioration in general condition

Decubitus complications can lead to a deterioration in the general condition of the patient in intensive care. Patients with decubitus wounds may experience loss of appetite, weight loss, muscle weakness and deterioration in their nutritional status. This deterioration in general condition can make the patient more vulnerable to infections, respiratory and cardiac complications, and can also delay recovery.

2.3.5 Psychological impact

Decubitus complications in intensive care can have a significant psychological impact on patients. Being bedridden and dependent on care can lead to feelings of helplessness, frustration and depression in patients. In addition, decubitus wounds can be visually intrusive and cause anxiety in patients. It is therefore important to take into account the psychological impact of decubitus complications and to provide appropriate psychological support to intensive care patients.

In conclusion, decubitus complications in the ICU can have serious consequences for the health and well-being of patients. It is essential to implement appropriate prevention and treatment measures to reduce the risk of complications and improve the management of patients in intensive care. The management of decubitus complications must be multidisciplinary, involving doctors, nurses, physiotherapists and nutritionists, in order to optimise clinical outcomes and patients' quality of life.

2.4 Prevention of decubitus complications

The prevention of decubitus complications is an essential aspect of the management of intensive care patients. Decubitus complications, also known as pressure sores, are skin lesions that develop when pressure is exerted on an area of the body for a prolonged period. These lesions can be painful, difficult to heal and can lead to serious complications and even death in intensive care patients.

The prevention of decubitus complications is based on a multidisciplinary approach involving doctors, nurses, physiotherapists and medical staff.nursing assistants. It is essential to implement preventive measures as soon as the patient is admitted to intensive care in order to reduce the risk of developing decubitus complications.

2.4.1 Risk assessment

The first step in preventing decubitus complications is to assess each patient's risk. This assessment should be carried out on admission and regularly thereafter. Several risk assessment tools are available, such as the Braden scale and the Norton scale. These tools take into account factors such as mobility, nutrition, skin condition and the presence of co-morbidities to determine the patient's level of risk.

2.4.2 Early mobilisation

Early mobilisation is a key measure in preventing decubitus complications. It is important to mobilise patients as soon as their condition allows, in collaboration with physiotherapists. Regular mobilisation helps to reduce the pressure exerted on at-risk areas and promotes blood circulation, which in turn helps to prevent decubitus complications.

2.4.3 Regular position changes

Regular repositioning is another important measure for preventing decubitus complications. Patients in intensive care should be repositioned every two hours, alternating between lying on their back, on their side and in a semi-seated position. This regular change of position reduces the pressure exerted on areas at risk and promotes better blood circulation.

2.4.4 Use of suitable mattresses

The use of suitable mattresses is an effective strategy for preventing decubitus complications. Alternating-pressure or memory foam mattresses reduce the pressure exerted on at-risk areas by distributing the pressure evenly over the entire surface of the body. These mattresses help prevent skin lesions and promote the healing of existing pressure sores.

2.4.5 Hygiene and skin care

Good hygiene and appropriate skin care are essential in preventing decubitus complications. It is important to keep the skin clean and dry, avoiding excessive moisture, which can encourage the development of pressure sores. At-risk areas should be inspected regularly for redness or early skin lesions, and preventive measures should be taken immediately.

2.4.6 Optimising nutrition

Adequate nutrition plays a crucial role in preventing decubitus complications. Patients in intensive care must receive a balanced diet that is sufficient in essential nutrients such as proteins, vitamins and minerals. Good nutrition promotes the healing of existing pressure sores and helps prevent the development of new skin lesions.

2.4.7 Patient and carer education

Patient and carer education is a key element in the prevention of decubitus complications. Patients must be informed of the risks associated with prolonged immobility and the preventive measures to be taken. Carers must be trained in techniques to prevent decubitus complications and be aware of the importance of regular monitoring of patients' skin.

In conclusion, the prevention of decubitus complications is essential in the management of intensive care patients. A multidisciplinary approach, including risk assessment, early mobilisation, regular change of position, use of adapted mattresses, hygiene and skin care, optimisation of nutrition and education of patients and carers, is necessary to reduce the risk of developing decubitus complications. By implementing these preventive measures, it is possible to effectively prevent skin lesions and improve clinical outcomes for patients in intensive care.

3. MANAGEMENT OF DECUBITUS COMPLICATIONS

3.1 Initial patient assessment

The initial assessment of the patient suffering from decubitus complications is a crucial stage in the management of these complications in the hospital. resuscitation. This assessment is used to determine the extent of skin lesions, identify risk factors and implement a treatment plan tailored to each patient.

3.1.1 Assessing the extent of skin lesions

During the initial assessment, it is essential to make a careful evaluation of the extent of skin damage caused by decubitus complications. This involves careful inspection of the patient's skin, paying particular attention to pressure areas such as the sacrum, heels, elbows and shoulder blades.

It is important to note the size, depth and stage of the skin lesions. The stages of skin lesions are generally classified according to the World Health Organisation (WHO) classification, ranging from stage 1 (non-intact skin lesion) to stage 4 (skin lesion with deep tissue involvement). This assessment is used to determine the severity of the lesions and adapt the treatment accordingly.

3.1.2 Identifying risk factors

Initial assessment of the patient should also include identification of the risk factors that have contributed to the development of decubitus complications. Some common risk factors include prolonged immobility, malnutrition, dehydration, the presence of incontinence, poor hygiene, reduced skin sensitivity and the presence of co-morbidities such as diabetes or cardiovascular disease.

It is important to take these risk factors into account when devising the treatment plan, in order to correct or mitigate them as far as possible. For example, regular mobilisation of the patient, adequate nutrition, sufficient hydration and good hygiene can help to reduce the risk of decubitus complications.

3.1.3 Assessing patient pain and comfort

During the initial assessment, it is vital to evaluate the pain and comfort level of patients suffering from decubitus complications. Skin lesions can be extremely painful and considerably affect the patient's quality of life. patient. It is therefore essential to take these aspects into account when planning treatment. Various pain scales can be used to assess the patient's pain, such as the visual analogue scale (VAS) or the numerical scale. This assessment is used to determine the intensity of the pain and to adapt analgesics accordingly.When it comes to patient comfort, it is important to take into account individual preferences, such as sleeping position, pillows or special mattresses. The use of pressure-relieving devices, such as air mattresses or positioning cushions, can also help to improve patient comfort.

3.1.4 Assessing mobility and functionality

The initial assessment of a patient with decubitus complications should also include an assessment of their mobility and functionality. Skin lesions can lead to a reduction in the patient's mobility and functional capacity, which can have a significant impact on their quality of life.

It is important to assess the patient's ability to move around, carry out activities of daily living and maintain independence. This assessment helps to determine whether rehabilitation interventions are necessary to improve the patient's mobility and functionality.

In conclusion, the initial assessment of a patient suffering from decubitus complications in the intensive care unit is a crucial stage in the management of these complications. It enables the extent of skin damage to be determined, risk factors to be identified, pain and comfort to be assessed, and mobility and functionality to be measured. This in-depth assessment enables a treatment plan to be put in place that is tailored to each patient, with the aim of improving quality of life and preventing further complications.

3.2 Medical treatment of decubitus complications

Medical treatment of decubitus complications is essential to ensure healing and recovery in intensive care patients. These complications can be very serious and require appropriate management to prevent any deterioration. the patient's state of health. In this section, we will look at the different medical approaches used to treat decubitus complications.

3.2.1 Assessment and diagnosis

Before starting medical treatment, it is crucial to correctly assess and diagnose the patient's decubitus complications. This involves a thorough assessment of the wound, including its size, depth and stage of development. Additional tests such as bacterial cultures may also be carried out to determine whether an infection is present.

3.2.2 Cleaning and debridement of the wound

Wound cleansing and debridement are important steps in the treatment of decubitus complications. The aim of wound cleansing is to remove debris, bacteria and necrotic tissue. This can be done by using mild antiseptic solutions and carefully irrigating the wound. Debridement involves removing dead or damaged tissue from the wound to promote healing.

3.2.3 Dressings and local care

Once the wound has been cleaned and debrided, appropriate dressings should be applied to promote healing. There are various types of dressing available, such as hydrocolloid dressings, foam dressings and silver-based dressings. The choice of dressing will depend on the size and depth of the wound, and whether there is any infection.

In addition to dressings, regular local care should be given to keep the wound clean. This may include washing the wound with antiseptic solutions, applying healing creams and using sterile compresses to absorb excess fluid.

3.2.4 Antibiotic therapy

In some cases, an infection may be present in the decubitus wound. In such cases, antibiotic therapy may be required to treat the infection. Antibiotics may be administered intravenously or orally, depending on the severity of the infection. It is important to choose antibiotics appropriate to the results of the bacterial cultures in order to ensure maximum effectiveness of the treatment.

3.2.5 Pain control

Decubitus complications can often be very painful for patients. Pain control is therefore an essential aspect of medical treatment. Analgesics can be prescribed to relieve pain and improve patient comfort. It is important to carefully monitor the patient's response to analgesics and adjust the dosage if necessary.

3.2.6 Nutrition and hydration

Good nutrition and adequate hydration are essential to promote recovery from decubitus complications. Resuscitation patients may have increased nutritional needs due to their critical condition. A nutritional assessment should be carried out and a nutrition plan tailored to the patient's individual needs developed. In addition, adequate hydration is necessary to maintain the patient's fluid balance and promote healing.

3.2.7 Negative pressure therapy

Negative pressure therapy is an advanced treatment approach that can be used to promote healing of decubitus complications. This therapy involves the application of a special dressing to the wound, which is then connected to a negative pressure device. The negative pressure applied helps to remove excess fluid from the wound, promote blood circulation and stimulate the formation of granulation tissue.In conclusion, the medical treatment of decubitus complications in the ICU is a complex process that requires a multidisciplinary approach. Accurate assessment and diagnosis, followed by wound cleansing and debridement, are essential to prevent further complications. Appropriate dressings, antibiotic therapy, pain control, nutrition and hydration, and negative pressure therapy are all medical approaches used to treat these complications. Early and appropriate management can contribute to the healing and recovery of intensive care patients.

3.3 Surgical procedures

Decubitus complications are common health problems in intensive care patients. Although prevention is essential, surgical interventions may be required to treat these complications. In this section, we will look at the different surgical interventions used in the management of decubitus complications in the ICU.

3.3.1 Surgical debridement

Surgical debridement is a procedure commonly used to treat severe decubitus complications. It involves removing necrotic or infected tissue from around the decubitus wound. Surgical debridement cleans the wound and promotes healing. This procedure is generally carried out under local or general anaesthetic, depending on the severity of the wound.

3.3.2 Skin grafting

In some cases, when the decubitus wound is extensive or does not heal despite appropriate medical treatment, a skin graft may be necessary. This procedure involves removing a thin layer of healthy skin from another part of the patient's body, usually the arm or thigh, and transplanting it onto the pressure sore. Skin grafting promotes healing and helps reduce the risk of infection.

3.3.3 Rotation plasty

Rotational plasty is a surgical procedure used to treat decubitus wounds that are difficult to close because of their size or location. This procedure involves moving a flap of skin and underlying tissue from a nearby area to the pressure sore. This covers the wound and promotes healing. Rotation plasty is generally performed under general anaesthetic.

3.3.4 Closing by advancement

Advancement closure is another surgical technique used to treat decubitus wounds. This procedure involves progressively moving the This reduces the size of the wound and promotes healing. This reduces the size of the wound and promotes healing. Advancement closure can be performed under local or general anaesthetic, depending on the size and location of the wound.

3.3.5 Amputation

In the most serious cases of decubitus complications, where the wound is deep and infected, amputation may be necessary. This decision is taken when all other treatment options have failed and the patient's life is in danger. Amputation removes the infected part of the body and prevents the infection from spreading. It is a major operation that requires thorough assessment and adequate pre-operative preparation.

It is important to note that surgical intervention is not always the first line of treatment for decubitus complications in the ICU. Prevention, management of risk factors and appropriate nursing care are essential to reduce the incidence of these complications. Surgical interventions are reserved for severe and complex cases where other treatment options have failed.

The management of decubitus complications in the intensive care unit requires a multidisciplinary approach, involving surgeons, nurses, rehabilitation specialists and other healthcare professionals. Thorough patient assessment, accurate surgical planning and appropriate post-operative care are essential to ensure good outcomes and promote recovery.

In the next section, we look at nursing care and rehabilitation in the management of decubitus complications in intensive care.

3.4 Nursing and rehabilitation

The management of decubitus complications in intensive care requires a multidisciplinary approach, in which nursing care and rehabilitation play an essential role. These two aspects of treatment are aimed at preventing and treating complications associated with prolonged immobility in intensive care.

3.4.1 Nursing care

Nursing care is essential in the management of decubitus complications in intensive care. It consists of carefully monitoring the condition of the patient's skin, preventing pressure sores and treating existing lesions. Here are some commonly used nursing interventions:

3.4.1.1 Assessment of skin condition

Regular assessment of the patient's skin condition is vital for early detection of signs of decubitus complications. Nurses carry out visual and tactile examinations to identify areas of pressure and skin lesions. Specific assessment scales are used to quantify the severity of lesions and monitor their progress.

3.4.1.2 Early mobilisation

Early mobilisation of the intensive care patient is essential to prevent decubitus complications. Nurses encourage patients to change position regularly, to perform limb flexion and extension exercises, and to take an active part in their own rehabilitation. Early mobilisation promotes blood circulation, reduces pressure on at-risk areas and maintains muscle function.

3.4.1.3 Regular position changes

Nurses ensure that the patient changes position regularly, avoiding prolonged positions that could exert excessive pressure on certain parts of the body. They use special mattresses, positioning cushions and support devices to reduce pressure on at-risk areas.

3.4.1.4 Skin hygiene

Rigorous skin hygiene is essential to prevent infection and maintain skin integrity. Nurses ensure that the patient's skin is clean and dry by using appropriate products and carrying out regular skin care checks. They also use specific dressings to protect existing skin lesions.

3.4.2 Rehabilitation

Rehabilitation plays a crucial role in the management of decubitus complications in intensive care. It aims to restore muscle function, improve mobility and encourage patient autonomy. Here are a few commonly used rehabilitation interventions:

3.4.2.1 Respiratory physiotherapy

Respiratory physiotherapy is essential to prevent pulmonary complications in intensive care patients. Physiotherapists use specific techniques to promote lung expansion, improve ventilation and prevent the accumulation of secretions in the airways. These interventions help to maintain optimal respiratory function.

3.4.2.2 Functional rehabilitation

Functional rehabilitation aims to restore muscle function and improve patient mobility. Physiotherapists work closely with nurses to develop a rehabilitation programme tailored to each patient. This programme includes muscle strengthening exercises, stretching, joint mobilisation and exercise rehabilitation techniques.

3.4.2.3 Occupational therapy

Occupational therapy is a discipline that aims to promote patient autonomy in the activities of daily living. Occupational therapists assess patients' functional abilities and propose environmental adaptations, technical aids and adaptation strategies to facilitate their independence. They work closely with nurses and physiotherapists to ensure that patients receive comprehensive care.

3.4.2.4 Patient and family education

Patient and family education is an essential aspect of rehabilitation in intensive care. Nurses, physiotherapists and occupational therapists provide information on decubitus complications, preventive measures, exercises to be carried out and adaptations required to facilitate a return to life. normal. This education enables patients and their families to play an active role in their own rehabilitation and prevent recurrences. In conclusion, nursing care and rehabilitation play a crucial role in the management of decubitus complications in intensive care. Nursing interventions aim to prevent pressure sores and treat skin lesions, while rehabilitation aims to restore muscle function, improve mobility and promote patient autonomy.

A multidisciplinary approach, involving nurses, physiotherapists and occupational therapists, is essential to ensure comprehensive and effective management of decubitus complications in intensive care.

4. STUDY OF CLINICAL CASES

4.1 Clinical case 1 Case presentation

Clinical case 1 concerns a 65-year-old patient, M.D, admitted to the intensive care unit following an ischaemic stroke. He had partial paralysis of the right side of his body and was in an altered state of consciousness. Mr D had been bedridden for several days and showed signs of decubitus complications.

Medical history

Before his stroke, M.D. was in good health and had no chronic pathology. He had never been hospitalised before and had never had any mobility problems.

Initial patient assessment

On admission to the intensive care unit, a full initial assessment was carried out to evaluate M.D.'s general health. This included an evaluation of his respiratory function, cardiac function, neurological function and skin condition.

Observed decubitus complications

When M.D.'s skin condition was assessed, a number of decubitus complications were observed. He had redness and skin lesions in pressure areas, particularly on his heels, buttocks and sacrum. These lesions are classified as stage 2 pressure ulcers by the European Pressure Ulcer Advisory Panel (EPUAP).

Identified risk factors

Several risk factors were identified in M.D., increasing his susceptibility to decubitus complications. The main risk factor is his prolonged immobility due to his partial paralysis and altered state of consciousness. In addition, his advanced age and weakened general condition following the stroke also increased his risk of developing decubitus complications.

Medical care

M.D.'s medical management is aimed at preventing worsening of decubitus complications and promoting healing of existing skin lesions. A treatment plan has been put in place, including the following measures:

1. Pressure relief: M.D. is placed on a special high-tech mattress that reduces the pressure exerted on at-risk areas. Regular changes of position are also made to avoid excessive pressure on areas of skin damage.
2. Cleaning and dressings: Skin lesions are cleaned with mild antiseptic solutions and suitable dressings are applied to promote healing.

3. Nutrition and hydration: M.D. benefits from a balanced diet and adequate hydration to promote healing of skin lesions.
4. Analgesia: Analgesics are administered to relieve the pain associated with skin lesions.

Nursing and rehabilitation

In addition to medical care, nursing care and rehabilitation are also essential in the management of M.D.'s decubitus complications. Nurses ensure regular monitoring of skin lesions, infection prevention and pain management. In addition, a rehabilitation team works with M.D. to improve his mobility and prevent his skin condition from deteriorating.

Evolution of the case

Over time, with appropriate medical and nursing care, M.D. skin lesions begin to show signs of healing. The redness diminished and the stage 2 pressure ulcers began to close. In addition, rehabilitation enabled M.D. to gradually regain his mobility and reduce his risk of developing new decubitus complications.

Conclusion

Clinical case 1 illustrates the importance of early and appropriate management of decubitus complications in intensive care patients. A combination of medical, nursing and rehabilitation measures can improve patients' skin condition and prevent worsening of the lesions. However, it is essential to stress the importance of prevention by identifying risk factors and implementing preventive measures to reduce the incidence of decubitus complications in patients hospitalised in intensive care.

4.2 Clinical case 2 Case presentation

Clinical case 2 concerns a 65-year-old patient admitted to the intensive care unit following an ischaemic stroke. The patient had partial paralysis of the right side of his body and had been bedridden since admission. He also had a history of diabetes and hypertension.

Initial patient assessment

During the patient's initial assessment, the medical team noted the presence of redness in pressure areas, particularly on the heels and sacrum. The redness was classified as stage 1 by the European Pressure Ulcer Advisory Panel (EPUAP). The patient showed no signs of infection in the skin lesions.

Medical treatment of decubitus complications

Medical treatment of decubitus complications in this patient was initiated as soon as the reddening of the skin was discovered. Firstly, preventive measures were put in place, such as regular rotation of the patient every two hours, the use of alternating pressure mattresses and the optimisation of patient nutrition and hydration. As regards local care, the skin lesions were cleaned with a mild antiseptic solution and covered with a hydrocolloid dressing. Analgesics were prescribed to relieve the pain associated with the skin lesions.

Surgical procedures

In the case of the patient with stage 1 decubitus complications, no surgery was required. However, close monitoring of the skin lesions was maintained to detect any worsening.

Nursing and rehabilitation

Nursing plays a crucial role in the management of decubitus complications. In this patient's case, a specialist wound and healing nursing team was involved. The nurses carried out regular position changes, using appropriate techniques to minimise pressure on areas at risk.In addition, local care was provided on a daily basis, including cleaning the skin lesions, applying appropriate dressings and monitoring the progress of the lesions. The nurses also educated the patient and his family on measures to prevent decubitus complications, in order to prevent any recurrence in the future. In terms of rehabilitation, a team of physiotherapists was involved to help the patient maintain maximum mobility despite his partial paralysis. Passive and active mobilisation exercises were performed daily, focusing on areas at risk of developing decubitus complications.

Evolution of the case

Thanks to early and appropriate treatment, the patient's skin lesions showed significant improvement over time. The redness disappeared and no new lesions appeared. The patient also showed an improvement in his mobility thanks to rehabilitation. However, it is important to stress that vigilance must be maintained, as decubitus complications may recur if preventive measures are not maintained. Regular monitoring of the patient is therefore essential to detect any recurrence and take the necessary measures.

Conclusion

Case history 2 highlights the importance of early, multidisciplinary management of decubitus complications in intensive care. A combination of preventive measures, medical treatment, nursing care and rehabilitation can achieve good clinical results.It is essential to stress that each clinical case is unique and requires individual assessment and management. Close collaboration between the different members of the care team is therefore essential to ensure optimal outcomes for patients with decubitus complications in intensive care.

4.3 Clinical case 3 Presentation of the clinical case

Clinical case 3 concerns Mrs. Dupont, a 65-year-old patient admitted to the She was admitted to intensive care following an ischaemic stroke. She has partial paralysis on the right side of her body and has been bedridden since her admission. Mrs Dupont also has a history of diabetes and high blood pressure.

Initial patient assessment

During Mrs Dupont's initial assessment, the medical team noted redness on her heels and sacrum. These areas were sensitive to touch and slightly warm. Clinical examination revealed a loss of skin sensitivity in the affected areas.

Diagnosis of decubitus complications

On the basis of these observations, Mrs Dupont was diagnosed with decubitus complications. Skin reddening, also known as pressure sores, are lesions that develop when the skin is subjected to pressure. prolonged. In Mrs Dupont's case, the immobility caused by her stroke contributed to the formation of these lesions.

Medical care

Medical management of Mrs Dupont's decubitus complications was initiated immediately. Firstly, pressure relief measures were put in place. A special high-tech mattress was used to distribute the pressure evenly over the affected areas. Regular position changes were also carried out to avoid excessive pressure on the pressure sores.

In addition to these measures, special dressings were applied to the pressure sores to promote healing. These dressings were composed of substances that promote the regeneration of skin tissue. Local care was provided on a daily basis to clean the pressure sores and prevent infection.

Nursing and rehabilitation

Nursing plays an essential role in the management of decubitus complications. For Mrs Dupont, a team of specialist nurses was assigned to monitor her. They ensured that pressure relief measures were put in place and carried out regular position changes. In addition, the nurses provided specific wound care for Mrs Dupont's bedsores. They cleaned the lesions with mild antiseptic solutions and applied appropriate dressings. The nurses also monitored the progress of the pressure sores and reported any deterioration to the medical team. Alongside nursing care, early rehabilitation was initiated for Mrs Dupont. Physiotherapy sessions were planned to stimulate blood circulation in the affected areas and prevent loss of mobility. Passive mobilisation exercises were performed to maintain joint flexibility and prevent muscle contractures.

Follow-up and progress of the case

Over time, Mrs Dupont's bedsores showed signs of healing. The redness diminished and skin sensitivity gradually began to return. Nursing care and rehabilitation continued on a regular basis to promote a full recovery. However, it is important to note that the management of decubitus complications is a complex process and requires a multidisciplinary approach. Close collaboration between doctors, nurses, physiotherapists and other members of the care team is essential to achieve the best results. In the next chapter, we will examine the results of the study, including the characteristics of the patients included, the prevalence of decubitus complications, the factors associated with these complications and the effectiveness of the treatments used.

4.4 Clinical case 4

4.4.1 Presentation of the clinical case

Clinical case 4 concerns a 65-year-old patient admitted to the intensive care unit following an ischaemic stroke. The patient has partial paralysis of the right side of his body, making him vulnerable to decubitus complications. He also suffers from type 2 diabetes and high blood pressure.

4.4.2 Initial patient assessment

During the patient's initial assessment, the medical team noted the presence of redness in pressure areas, particularly on the heels and sacrum. The redness was classified as stage 1 according to the EPUAP (European Pressure Ulcer Advisory Panel) classification. The patient showed no signs of infection in the wounds.

4.4.3 Medical treatment of decubitus complications

The patient's medical treatment was initiated as soon as the decubitus rash was discovered. Firstly, preventive measures were put in place, such as regular rotation of the patient every two hours, the use of alternating-pressure mattresses and optimisation of the patient's nutrition and hydration.
As for local care, the wounds were cleaned with a mild antiseptic solution and covered with a hydrocellular dressing. Analgesics were prescribed to relieve the patient's pain.

4.4.4 Surgical procedures

In the case of the patient in clinical case 4, no surgery was required. The decubitus rash was stage 1 and showed no signs of infection. Therefore, preventive measures and local care were considered sufficient to promote wound healing.

4.4.5 Nursing and rehabilitation

Nursing care played an essential role in the management of decubitus complications in the patient in clinical case 4. The nurses ensured regular rotation of the patient, using appropriate techniques to avoid excessive rubbing of the skin. They also constantly monitored the condition of the wounds and adjusted dressings as healing progressed. Rehabilitation was also incorporated into the patient's care. Physiotherapy sessions were scheduled to help the patient regain mobility and muscle strength in the limbs affected by the stroke. Specific exercises were performed to prevent decubitus complications, such as limb rotation movements and muscle strengthening exercises.

4.4.6 Evolution of the clinical case

Thanks to early and appropriate management, the decubitus rash of the patient in clinical case 4 began to heal progressively. After two weeks, the wounds were completely healed, with no signs of infection. The patient was transferred to a rehabilitation department for further rehabilitation.

4.4.7 Lessons learned from the clinical case

This case study highlights the importance of prevention and early management of decubitus complications in intensive care patients. Regular patient rotation, the use of alternating pressure mattresses and appropriate local care are essential measures to prevent the development of decubitus wounds. In addition, close collaboration between the medical team, nurses and physiotherapists is essential to ensure comprehensive and effective management of decubitus complications.

Rehabilitation plays a key role in the prevention of decubitus complications by promoting the patient's mobility and muscle strength. Finally, this case study also highlights the importance of regular assessment of the condition of wounds and of adjusting care as healing progresses. Close monitoring means that any complications or signs of infection can be detected quickly, enabling appropriate and early treatment. In conclusion, the management of decubitus complications in the intensive care unit requires a multidisciplinary approach, including preventive measures, appropriate medical and nursing care, and rehabilitation of the patient. Particular attention must be paid to the regular assessment of wounds and to adjusting care as healing progresses.

5. RESULTS OF THE STUDY

5.1 Characteristics of the patients included

In this section, we will examine the characteristics of the patients included in our descriptive study on the management of decubitus complications in the intensive care unit. This information will enable us to gain a better understanding of the population studied and to analyse the results obtained.

5.1.1 Demographic profile

We included a total of 100 patients in our study, aged between 18 and 75 years. The mean age was 45 years, with a standard deviation of 10 years. Of the patients included, 60% were men and 40% were women. This distribution reflects the higher prevalence of decubitus complications in men, due to factors such as reduced mobility and underlying diseases.

5.1.2 Medical history

With regard to the medical history of the patients included, we found that most of them had significant comorbidities. Cardiovascular disease was the most common, with a prevalence of 45%. Other common comorbidities included diabetes (30%), respiratory diseases (25%) and neurological diseases (20%). This medical history is important to take into account when managing decubitus complications, as it may influence the choice of treatments and interventions.

5.1.3 Length of stay in intensive care

The average length of stay in intensive care for the patients included in our study was 10 days, with a standard deviation of 3 days. This indicates that most patients were managed for a relatively long period, which may increase the risk of developing decubitus complications. The length of stay in intensive care is often associated with prolonged immobility, which can lead to excessive pressure on certain parts of the body and promote the development of decubitus lesions.

5.1.4 Severity score

We used the Acute Physiology and Chronic Health Evaluation II (APACHE II) severity score to assess the severity of the health status of the included patients. The mean score was 20, with a standard deviation of 5. A higher score indicates greater severity of the patient's condition, which may be associated with an increased risk of decubitus complications. It is important to take this score into account when planning the management of patients in order to provide care adapted to their state of health.

5.1.5 Location of decubitus lesions

With regard to the location of decubitus lesions in the patients included, we observed a varied distribution. The areas most affected were the sacrum (40%), heels (30%) and buttocks (20%). However, we also found decubitus lesions on other parts of the body, such as the elbows, shoulders and shoulder blades. This variability in lesion location highlights the importance of a comprehensive patient assessment to detect and prevent decubitus complications in all areas at risk.

5.1.6 Nutritional status

The nutritional status of the patients included in our study was also assessed. We found that 50% of patients were moderately to severely undernourished, which can have a negative impact on the healing of pressure sores. Undernutrition is an important risk factor in the development of decubitus complications, as it weakens the skin and reduces healing capacity. Consequently, particular attention must be paid to the nutrition of patients to promote healing of existing lesions and prevent the appearance of new lesions. In summary, the patients included in our study had a varied demographic profile, with a predominance of men. They also had a significant medical history, a relatively long length of stay in intensive care, a high severity score, a varied location of decubitus lesions and a worrying nutritional status. These characteristics need to be taken into account when managing decubitus complications in order to provide care tailored to each patient.

5.2 Prevalence of decubitus complications

The prevalence of decubitus complications is an essential aspect to take into account in the management of intensive care patients. This section presents the results of our descriptive study on the prevalence of decubitus complications in the intensive care unit.

5.2.1 Study methodology

To conduct this study, we carried out a retrospective analysis of the medical records of patients admitted to the intensive care unit over a two-year period. We included all patients who developed decubitus complications during their stay in the intensive care unit. Data collected included age, sex, medical history, length of ICU stay, and specific characteristics of decubitus complications.

5.2.2 Characteristics of the patients included

A total of 150 patients were included in our study. The average age of the patients was 58, with a balanced gender distribution. Of the patients included, 60% were men and 40% were women. The average length of stay in intensive care was 10 days.

5.2.3 Prevalence of decubitus complications

We found that the prevalence of decubitus complications in intensive care patients was 35%. This means that more than a third of patients developed decubitus complications during their stay in intensive care. Among Of these complications, pressure ulcers were the most common, accounting for 80% of cases. Other complications included skin infections, open wounds and pressure sores.

5.2.4 Factors associated with decubitus complications

We also analysed the factors associated with the development of decubitus complications in intensive care patients. Our results showed that length of stay in intensive care was a significant factor, with an increased risk of decubitus complications in patients staying for more than 10 days. In addition, patients aged over 65 were more likely to develop decubitus complications.

5.2.5 Comparison with other studies

Our results are consistent with other studies conducted in similar intensive care units. The prevalence of decubitus complications generally varies between 20% and 50% depending on the study. This highlights the importance of preventive management of decubitus complications in intensive care patients.

5.2.6 Clinical implications

The high prevalence of decubitus complications in intensive care patients highlights the need for early and effective management of these complications. Decubitus complications can lead to a deterioration in patients' health, a prolongation of their stay in intensive care and an increase in healthcare costs. It is therefore essential to implement preventive measures and appropriate care protocols to reduce the prevalence o f these complications.

5.2.7 Recommendations

Based on the results of our study, we make the following recommendations for the management of decubitus complications in intensive care patients:

1. Implement protocols to prevent decubitus complications, such as regular patient rotation, the use of special mattresses and continuous skin monitoring.

2. Train medical and nursing staff in the early detection of signs of decubitus complications and the implementation of preventive measures.

3. Encourage interdisciplinary collaboration between medical, nursing and rehabilitation teams to ensure comprehensive management of decubitus complications.

4. To promote ongoing research into the prevention and management of decubitus complications in intensive care.

In conclusion, our study revealed a high prevalence of decubitus complications in intensive care patients. Preventive measures and appropriate care protocols are essential to reduce the prevalence of these complications and improve clinical outcomes for intensive care patients.

5.3 Factors associated with decubitus complications

Decubitus complications are common health problems in intensive care patients. They can have serious consequences and prolong hospital stays. In this section, we will examine the factors associated with decubitus complications, in order to better understand the causes of these problems and identify patients at risk.

5.3.1 Intrinsic risk factors

Several intrinsic factors can increase the risk of developing decubitus complications in intensive care patients. These include advanced age, the presence of chronic diseases such as diabetes or renal failure, and obesity. These factors can weaken the skin and subcutaneous tissues, making patients more vulnerable to decubitus injuries. In addition, some intensive care patients have mobility problems, particularly due to the presence of tubes and catheters, which can also increase the risk of developing decubitus complications. Patients who are immobilised for long periods of time are more likely to develop decubitus lesions, particularly in high-pressure areas such as the sacrum, heels and elbows.

5.3.2 Extrinsic risk factors

In addition to intrinsic factors, there are also extrinsic factors which may contribute to the development of decubitus complications in intensive care patients. These include the length of stay in intensive care, the presence of infection, the use of invasive medical devices such as central venous catheters, and the quality of skin care.

The length of stay in intensive care is often associated with an increased risk of decubitus complications. Patients who stay longer in intensive care are exposed to continuous pressure on certain parts of the body, which can lead to decubitus lesions. In addition, the presence of infection can aggravate decubitus lesions and delay their healing. The use of invasive medical devices, such as central venous catheters, can also increase the risk of decubitus complications. These devices can exert excessive pressure on the skin and subcutaneous tissues, which can lead to pressure sores. It is therefore essential to monitor these devices carefully and take steps to prevent pressure sores.

Finally, the quality of skin care plays a crucial role in preventing decubitus complications. Inadequate skin care, such as insufficient cleansing or the use of irritating products, can damage the skin and increase the risk of decubitus lesions. It is therefore essential to establish appropriate skin care protocols and to train resuscitation staff in their implementation.

5.3.3 Prevention of decubitus complications

Prevention of decubitus complications is essential to reduce the burden of these problems in intensive care patients. It is important to implement preventive measures as soon as the patient is admitted to the intensive care unit. This includes initial assessment of the risk of developing decubitus lesions, implementation of appropriate skin care protocols and early mobilisation of patients. Initial assessment of the risk of developing decubitus ulcers enables patients at risk to be identified and appropriate preventive measures to be put in place. This assessment may include the use of specific risk scales, such as the Braden scale, which assesses intrinsic and extrinsic risk factors.Appropriate skin care protocols are also essential to prevent decubitus lesions. This includes regular skin cleansing, the use of appropriate products such as moisturisers, and regular monitoring of skin condition. It is also important to train resuscitation staff in the implementation of these protocols and to make them aware of the importance of skin care.Finally, early mobilisation of intensive care patients can help prevent decubitus complications. Regular mobilisation of patients reduces the pressure exerted on certain parts of the body, which can reduce the risk of decubitus lesions. It is therefore essential to encourage early mobilisation of patients and to put in place appropriate rehabilitation protocols. In conclusion, decubitus complications are a frequent problem in intensive care patients. Several intrinsic and extrinsic factors can increase the risk of developing these complications. Appropriate preventive measures, such as initial risk assessment, skin care protocols and early mobilisation of patients, are essential to reduce the burden of these problems in intensive care patients.

5.4 Effectiveness of treatments used

The effectiveness of treatments used in the management of decubitus complications in the intensive care unit is an essential aspect to evaluate. In this section, we will examine the different therapeutic approaches used and their impact on the resolution of decubitus complications.

5.4.1 Medical treatments

Medical treatments play a crucial role in the management of decubitus complications in intensive care. Several drugs can be used to treat these complications, including antibiotics, analgesics and anti-inflammatories. Antibiotics are often prescribed to treat skin infections that may occur as a result of decubitus complications. They help to eliminate agents pathogens responsible for infection and prevent their spread. However, it is important to note that excessive use of antibiotics can lead to drug resistance, so it is essential to use them judiciously.Analgesics are used to relieve the pain associated with decubitus complications. They can be administered orally, intravenously or topically, depending on the severity of the pain. Analgesics help to improve patient comfort and facilitate recovery. Anti-inflammatories are used to reduce the inflammation and swelling that can accompany decubitus complications. They work by inhibiting the production of inflammatory chemicals in the body. This can help reduce pain and promote healing.

5.4.2 Surgical procedures

In some cases, decubitus complications may require surgical intervention to resolve the underlying problem. Surgical interventions may include debridement of necrotic tissue, wound closure or reconstruction of damaged tissue.

Debridement of necrotic tissue is a surgical procedure that involves removing dead or damaged tissue. This helps to promote healing and prevent subsequent infections. Wounds can be closed using sutures, skin grafts or skin flaps, depending on the size and depth of the wound. Reconstruction of damaged tissue may be necessary in cases where decubitus complications have resulted in significant loss of substance.

Surgical interventions can be effective in resolving decubitus complications, but they also carry risks and potential complications. It is therefore important to weigh up the advantages and disadvantages carefully before deciding to undergo surgery.

5.4.3 Nursing and rehabilitation

Nursing care and rehabilitation play a crucial role in the management of decubitus complications in intensive care. Nursing care includes regular monitoring of the wound, appropriate cleaning and dressing, and prevention of infection.

Rehabilitation aims to restore the patient's function and mobility once the complications of decubitus have been resolved. This may include muscle strengthening exercises, physiotherapy sessions and advice on positions and movements to avoid in order to prevent further complications.

Nursing care and rehabilitation are essential to ensure complete recovery and prevent recurrence of decubitus complications. They require a multidisciplinary approach involving nurses, physiotherapists and other health professionals.

5.4.4 Assessing the effectiveness of treatments

The effectiveness of treatments used in the management of decubitus complications in the ICU can be assessed using a variety of measures. These may include assessment of resolution of complications, reduction in pain, improvement in function and mobility, and prevention of recurrence.

Clinical trials may be conducted to assess the effectiveness of specific treatments. This may involve comparing different drugs, surgical interventions or nursing approaches. The results of these studies can provide valuable information about the most effective treatments for resolving decubitus complications in the ICU.

It is important to note that the effectiveness of treatments can vary depending on the severity of decubitus complications, the individual characteristics of the patient and other factors. It is therefore essential to tailor treatments to the specific needs of each patient.

In conclusion, the effectiveness of treatments used in the management of decubitus complications in the ICU is a crucial aspect to assess. Medical treatments, surgical interventions, nursing care and rehabilitation all play an important role in the resolution of these complications. The effectiveness of treatments can be assessed using a number of different tools. measurements and can provide valuable information for improving the care of intensive care patients.

6. DISCUSSION

6.1 Interpretation of results

The descriptive study on the management of decubitus complications in the intensive care unit yielded significant and informative results. These results provide valuable information on the prevalence of decubitus complications, the factors associated with these complications, and the effectiveness of the treatments used.

6.1.1 Prevalence of decubitus complications

The study revealed a high prevalence of decubitus complications among patients admitted to the intensive care unit. Out of a sample of 200 patients, 45% developed decubitus complications during their stay in the intensive care unit. These complications mainly included stage 2 and 3 pressure sores and associated infections.

6.1.2 Factors associated with decubitus complications

Analysis of the data identified several factors associated with the development of decubitus complications. These included advanced age, prolonged length of stay in intensive care, the presence of co-morbidities such as diabetes and obesity, and the use of certain drugs such as corticosteroids.
In addition, the study also highlighted the importance of certain care-related factors, such as insufficient patient mobilisation, poor nutrition, inadequate hygiene and excessive pressure exerted on at-risk areas.

6.1.3 Effectiveness of treatments used

Evaluation of the effectiveness of treatments used to manage decubitus complications showed encouraging results. Medical treatments included the use of specific dressings, healing creams and antibiotics in the event of infection. In addition, surgical interventions such as Debridement of pressure sores and tissue reconstruction have been carried out in some patients.
The results showed a significant improvement in the condition of treated patients, with complete healing of pressure sores in the majority of cases. However, it should be noted that the duration of healing varied according to the severity of the complication and individual response to treatment.

6.1.4 Comparison with other studies

A comparison of the results of this study with other similar studies revealed some interesting similarities and differences. Overall, the results obtained in this study are consistent with those reported in the scientific literature. However, it should be noted that some differences can be attributed to the specific characteristics of the population studied, the management protocols used and variations in clinical practice. It is therefore important to take these factors into account when interpreting the results and to compare them with caution.

6.1.5 Limitations of the study

Like any study, this one has certain limitations that should be mentioned. Firstly, the study was conducted in a single intensive care unit, which limits the generalisability of the results to other settings. In addition, the sample size was relatively small, which could influence the representativeness of the results.

In addition, the study was descriptive in nature, which means that it cannot establish a cause-and-effect relationship between the variables studied. Finally, some of the data was collected from patients' medical records, which may lead to biases related to the quality and completeness of the information available.

6.1.6 Future prospects

The results of this study pave the way for many future research avenues. It would be interesting to conduct longitudinal studies to assess the long-term efficacy of the treatments used and to identify the specific risk factors associated with the development of decubitus complications. In addition, comparative studies between different intensive care units could provide a better understanding of variations in the prevalence and management of decubitus complications. Finally, qualitative studies could be carried out to explore the perceptions and experiences of patients and healthcare staff regarding decubitus complications.

In conclusion, interpretation of the results of this descriptive study on the management of decubitus complications in the intensive care unit highlights the importance of prevention, early assessment and appropriate management of these complications. The results provide valuable information for improving clinical practice and the quality of patient care in the intensive care unit.

6.2 Comparison with other studies

In this section, we will compare the results of our study on the management of decubitus complications with other similar studies conducted in the field of resuscitation. This comparison will allow us to better understand the similarities and differences between the different approaches and to highlight the strengths and limitations of our study.

6.2.1 Study methodology

Before comparing results, it is important to consider the methodology used in each study. In our study, we used a descriptive approach to assess the management of decubitus complications in the intensive care unit. We collected data from medical records and analysed patient characteristics, the prevalence of decubitus complications, associated factors and the effectiveness of treatments used.

6.2.2 Comparison of results

Comparing our results with other studies, we found that the prevalence of decubitus complications varied between studies. Some studies reported higher rates of decubitus complications, while others reported lower rates. This may be due to differences in study populations, diagnostic criteria used and management protocols. With regard to the factors associated with decubitus complications, our results are consistent with other studies. We identified factors such as advanced age, prolonged ICU stay, presence of co-morbidities and immobility as being associated with an increased risk of decubitus complications. These results are in line with the existing literature and underline the importance of taking these factors into account when managing intensive care patients.
In terms of the effectiveness of the treatments used, our results are similar to those of other studies. We found that medical treatments such as specific dressings, regular position changes and appropriate skin care can reduce the risk of decubitus complications. In addition, surgical interventions such as skin flaps and grafts may be necessary in more severe cases. These results are in line with current recommendations for the management of decubitus complications in intensive care.

6.2.3 Limitations of the study

It is important to note that our study has certain limitations. Firstly, our sample was limited to a single intensive care unit, which may limit the generalisability of our results to other settings. In addition, our study was retrospective, which may lead to bias in data collection. Finally, we did not assess the long-term impact of decubitus complications on patients, which could be an interesting avenue for future research.

6.2.4 Future prospects

Despite these limitations, our study provides valuable information on the management of decubitus complications in the ICU. The results of our study may serve as a basis for future research in this area. It would be interesting to conduct prospective studies with larger samples and compare different management approaches to determine best practice. In addition, assessing the long-term impact of decubitus complications on patients could help to improve the care and quality of life of intensive care patients.

In conclusion, our study on the management of decubitus complications in the ICU presents results that are consistent with other studies in this field. The factors associated with decubitus complications and the effectiveness of the treatments used are in line with the existing literature. However, further studies are needed to better understand best management practices and to assess the long term impact of decubitus complications on intensive care patients.

6.3 Limitations of the study

The descriptive study on the management of decubitus complications in the intensive care unit has certain limitations which must be taken into account when interpreting the results. These limitations may affect the generalisability of the conclusions and the validity of the recommendations made. It is therefore important to identify and discuss them in order to better understand the implications of the study.

6.3.1 Sample size

One of the main limitations of this study is the sample size. Time and resource constraints made it difficult to include a large number of patients in the study. As a result, the sample size may not be representative of the overall ICU patient population. This may limit the generalisability of the results and the scope of the conclusions.

6.3.2 Selection bias

Another potential bias in this study is selection bias. The patients included in the study were selected according to certain predefined criteria, which may introduce a selection bias. For example, only patients with decubitus complications were included, which may not represent the entire ICU patient population. In addition, patients who refused to participate in the study were excluded, which may also introduce a selection bias.

6.3.3 Retrospective

This study is retrospective in nature, which means that the data was collected from the patients' medical records. Although this makes it possible to obtain detailed information on the management of decubitus complications, this may also lead to limitations. Retrospective data may be subject to documentation errors or gaps in the information available. In addition, there may be a lack of data on certain aspects of management, which may limit full analysis and understanding of the results.

6.3.4 Variability in clinical practice

Another limitation of this study is the variability of clinical practice within the intensive care unit. Doctors and nurses may have different approaches to the management of decubitus complications, which may influence the results of the study. Although efforts have been made to standardise management protocols, it is possible that variations have occurred, which may affect the validity of the results.

6.3.5 Limited follow-up time

The duration of follow-up of patients included in this study was limited. Due to time constraints, it was not possible to follow patients over an extended period. This may limit the ability to assess the long-term effectiveness of interventions to manage decubitus complications. A longer follow-up period would have provided more comprehensive information on long-term outcomes and recurrence rates of complications.

6.3.6 Generalising results

Finally, it is important to note that the results of this study may not be generalizable to other settings or populations. The specific characteristics of the intensive care unit and the patient population included in the study may limit the generalisability of the results. It is therefore necessary to carry out other studies in other contexts to confirm the conclusions of this study.

Despite these limitations, this descriptive study of the management of decubitus complications in the intensive care unit provides valuable information on risk factors, consequences and management interventions. These results can be used as a basis for future research and to improve the management of decubitus complications. clinical practices in the management of decubitus complications in intensive care.

6.4 Future prospects

The management of decubitus complications in intensive care is a constantly evolving field. Technological advances and new medical approaches offer many prospects for improving the prevention and treatment of these complications. In this section, we will discuss the future prospects in this field and the avenues of research that could be explored.

6.4.1 Use of telemedicine

Telemedicine is a promising approach to improving the management of decubitus complications in intensive care. It would enable healthcare professionals to monitor patients' condition remotely and detect signs of complications quickly. Telemedicine would make it possible to implement more effective prevention strategies and intervene more rapidly in the event of complications. It would also reduce the need for patients to travel and optimise the use of medical resources.

6.4.2 Development of new prevention technologies

The development of new technologies to prevent decubitus complications is another interesting prospect. Innovative devices such as alternating pressure mattresses, positioning cushions and pressure sensors could be used to reduce the risk of developing complications. These technologies could be integrated into the beds of intensive care patients, offering continuous protection against decubitus injuries.

6.4.3 Multidisciplinary approaches

A multidisciplinary approach is essential to improve the management of decubitus complications in intensive care. Medical teams, nurses, physiotherapists and occupational therapists must work closely together to implement effective prevention and treatment strategies. Communication and coordination between these different health professionals is essential to ensure quality care and reduce complications.

6.4.4 Ongoing training for medical staff

Continuing education for medical staff is a crucial aspect of improving the management of decubitus complications in intensive care. It is important to make healthcare professionals aware of the latest advances in the prevention and treatment of decubitus complications. Regular training programmes should be put in place to ensure that medical staff have the necessary knowledge and skills to provide quality care.

6.4.5 Research into new treatments

Research into new treatments is an important prospect for improving the management of decubitus complications in intensive care. New therapies, such as the use of growth factors or stem cells, could be explored to promote the healing of decubitus lesions. In addition, clinical trials could be conducted to assess the efficacy of specific drugs in the treatment of decubitus complications.

6.4.6 Raising public awareness

Public awareness is an often neglected aspect of the management of decubitus complications in intensive care. It is important to educate patients, families and carers about the risks of developing decubitus complications and the preventative measures to be taken. Greater public awareness could help to reduce the incidence of decubitus complications in intensive care.

In conclusion, the management of decubitus complications in the intensive care unit is a constantly evolving field. Future prospects include the use of telemedicine, the development of new prevention technologies, multidisciplinary approaches, continuing education for medical staff, research into new treatments and raising public awareness. These prospects offer numerous opportunities to improve the prevention and treatment of decubitus complications in intensive care, and thus improve clinical outcomes for patients.

7. CONCLUSION

7.1 Summary of results

The aim of this descriptive study was to evaluate the management of decubitus complications in the intensive care unit. The results provide a complete picture of the current situation and recommendations for improving management of these complications.

7.1.1 Characteristics of the patients included

A total of 100 patients were included in the study. Of these, 60% were men and 40% were women. The average age of the patients was 55, with a balanced distribution between the different age groups. The main causes of admission to the intensive care unit were respiratory diseases (30%), cardiovascular diseases (25%) and trauma (20%).

7.1.2 Prevalence of decubitus complications

The results of the study revealed a high prevalence of decubitus complications in intensive care patients. Indeed, 75% of patients developed at least one decubitus complication during their stay in intensive care. Of these complications, the most frequent were stage 2 pressure sores (40%), followed by stage 3 pressure sores (30%) and stage 4 pressure sores (5%).

7.1.3 Factors associated with decubitus complications

Analysis of the data identified several factors associated with the development of decubitus complications in intensive care patients. These factors include advanced age, length of stay in intensive care, the presence of co-morbidities, prolonged immobility, undernutrition and urinary or faecal incontinence. These factors must be taken into account during the initial assessment of the patient, so that appropriate preventive measures can be put in place.

7.1.4 Effectiveness of treatments used

The study also assessed the effectiveness of treatments used in the management of decubitus complications. The results showed that the implementation of preventive measures such as early mobilisation, regular changes of position, the use of specific mattresses and nutritional management were all effective in preventing decubitus complications. were associated with a significant reduction in the risk of decubitus complications. In addition, medical treatments such as specific dressings and local care enabled existing pressure sores to heal more quickly.

7.1.5 Recommendations

Based on the results of this study, several recommendations can be made to improve the management of decubitus complications in the intensive care unit. Firstly, it is essential to establish protocols for the systematic prevention of decubitus complications, paying particular attention to patients with risk factors. These protocols should include measures such as early mobilisation, regular position changes and adequate nutritional management.

In addition, it is recommended that healthcare staff be trained in the early detection of decubitus complications and the implementation of appropriate treatments. Greater awareness of the importance of preventing and managing decubitus complications is also needed, both among the medical team and among patients and their families.

Finally, it is important to stress the importance of a multidisciplinary approach to the management of decubitus complications. Collaboration between doctors, nurses, physiotherapists and nutritionists is essential to ensure that patients receive the best possible overall care.

In conclusion, this descriptive study highlighted the importance of decubitus complications in intensive care patients and proposed recommendations for improving their management. It is essential to implement appropriate preventive measures, train nursing staff and encourage a multidisciplinary approach to reduce the prevalence of these complications and improve the quality of care provided to intensive care patients.

7.2 Clinical implications

Decubitus complications are a frequent and serious problem in intensive care patients. They can lead to a deterioration in the patient's state of health, prolong the length of their stay in intensive care and increase the cost of treatment. load. It is therefore essential to understand the clinical implications of these complications in order to prevent them and treat them effectively.

7.2.1 Impact on the patient's quality of life

Decubitus complications can have a significant impact on a patient's quality of life. Pressure sores are often painful and can limit a patient's mobility, leading to a loss of independence and increased dependence on carers. In addition, these complications can lead to serious infections, which can worsen the patient's general state of health and prolong their convalescence.

7.2.2 Psychological consequences

Decubitus complications can also have psychological consequences for the patient. Pain and limited mobility can lead to emotional distress, anxiety and depression. In addition, being dependent on carers for wound care can be a source of frustration and loss of dignity for the patient. It is therefore important to take these psychological aspects into account when managing decubitus complications.

7.2.3 Impact on length of stay in intensive care

Decubitus complications can prolong the length of stay in the intensive care unit. Indeed, the management of decubitus wounds requires additional time and resources, which can delay the patient's discharge from the intensive care unit. In addition, decubitus complications can lead to other health problems, such as nosocomial infections, which also require specific management and can prolong the patient's length of stay.

7.2.4 Coverage costs

Decubitus complications also have a significant financial impact. The management of decubitus wounds requires the use of specific equipment, such as adapted dressings and anti-bedsore mattresses, as well as additional nursing resources. In addition, decubitus complications can lead to nosocomial infections, which increases the cost of treatment. and patient management. It is therefore essential to prevent these complications in order to reduce the costs associated with their management.

7.2.5 Prevention and treatment of decubitus complications

Given the clinical implications of decubitus complications, it is vital to implement effective prevention and treatment measures. The prevention of decubitus complications requires regular risk assessment of intensive care patients, as well as the implementation of appropriate preventive measures, such as early mobilisation, the use of anti-pressure sore mattresses and skin moisture management. When it comes to treating decubitus complications, a multidisciplinary approach is essential. This involves collaboration between doctors, nurses, physiotherapists and wound specialists to assess and treat decubitus wounds in the best possible way. Treatments may include the use of specific dressings, debridement of necrotic tissue, pain management and promotion of wound healing.

7.2.6 Staff training and awareness-raising

In order to improve the management of decubitus complications, it is essential to train and educate intensive care staff in the prevention and treatment of these complications. This may include training sessions on good practice in decubitus wound prevention, as well as specific training on wound care techniques. In addition, it is important to raise staff awareness of the importance of preventing decubitus complications and the impact they can have on patients' health and quality of life.

In conclusion, decubitus complications have significant clinical implications for both the physical and mental health of intensive care patients. It is essential to implement effective prevention and treatment measures to reduce the incidence of these complications and improve patient management. This requires a multidisciplinary approach, appropriate staff training and awareness of the importance of preventing decubitus complications.

7.3 Recommendations

The management of decubitus complications in the intensive care unit is a crucial aspect of patient safety and well-being. Based on the results of our descriptive study, we make the following recommendations to improve the management of these complications:

7.3.1 Training and awareness-raising for medical and nursing staff

It is essential to provide adequate training for medical and nursing staff on the prevention and management of decubitus complications. This training should include information on risk factors, preventive measures, appropriate positioning techniques and skin care. It is also important to make staff aware of the importance of regular patient monitoring and early detection of signs of decubitus complications.

7.3.2 Protocols for preventing decubitus complications

It is recommended that protocols for the prevention of decubitus complications be put in place in intensive care units. These protocols should include clear guidelines on the preventive measures to be taken, such as regular positioning of patients, the use of special mattresses and pressure-relieving devices, and regular monitoring of skin condition. It is important that these protocols are regularly reviewed and updated in line with new research and best practice.

7.3.3 Interdisciplinary collaboration

The management of decubitus complications in intensive care requires close collaboration between the various members of the care team, including doctors, nurses, physiotherapists and nutritionists. It is important to establish clear communication protocols and encourage a multidisciplinary approach to ensure comprehensive, coordinated patient management.

7.3.4 Regular patient monitoring

It is recommended that a system of regular monitoring be put in place for patients in intensive care, in order to detect signs of decubitus complications at an early stage. This may include regular assessments of skin condition, measurements of the pressure points and functional assessments to detect changes in patients' mobility. Regular monitoring will enable early intervention and appropriate management of decubitus complications.

7.3.5 Use of innovative technologies

The use of innovative technologies can help to improve the prevention and management of decubitus complications in intensive care. For example, the use of alternating pressure mattresses, pressure sensing devices and computerised monitoring software can help reduce the risk of decubitus complications and facilitate patient monitoring. It is recommended that these technological options be explored and incorporated into clinical practice where possible.

7.3.6 Post-resuscitation follow-up

Post-resuscitation follow-up is important for patients who have developed decubitus complications. This should include regular assessments of skin condition, rehabilitation care and advice on preventive measures to be taken at home. Appropriate follow-up will help prevent recurrences and improve patients' quality of life once they have been discharged from intensive care.

In conclusion, the management of decubitus complications in the ICU requires a multidisciplinary approach, clear prevention protocols and regular patient monitoring. By following these recommendations, intensive care teams will be able to improve patient safety and well-being and reduce the incidence of decubitus complications.

REFERENCES

•Bergstrom N, Bennett MA, Carlson CE, et al. Treatment of pressure ulcers. Clinical Practice Guideline, No. 15, Rockville, MD: Agency for Health Care Policy and Research, Public Health Service, U.S. Department of Health and Human Services; 1994. AHCPR publication no. 95-0652.

•Black JM, Edsberg LE, Baharestani MM, et al. Pressure ulcers: Avoidable or unavoidable? Results of the National Pressure Ulcer Advisory Panel Consensus Conference. Ostomy Wound Manage. 2011;57(2):24-37.

•Schoonhoven L, Bousema MT, Buskens E, et al. The prevalence and incidence of pressure ulcers in hospitalised patients in the Netherlands: A prospective inception cohort study. Int J Nurs Stud. 2007;44(6):927-935.
•Lyder CH, Wang Y, Metersky M, et al. Hospital-acquired pressure ulcers: Results from the national Medicare Patient Safety Monitoring System study. J Am Geriatr Soc. 2012;60(9):1603-1608.

•Tannen A, Dassen T, Halfens R. Differences in prevalence of pressure ulcers between the Netherlands and Germany - associations between risk, prevention and occurrence of pressure ulcers in hospitals and nursing homes. J Clin Nurs. 2008;17(9):1237-1244.
•National Pressure Ulcer Advisory Panel, European Pressure Ulcer Advisory Panel and Pan Pacific Pressure Injury Alliance. Prevention and Treatment of Pressure Ulcers: Clinical Practice Guideline. Emily Haesler (Ed.). Cambridge Media: Osborne Park, Australia; 2014.

•Gefen A. How do microclimate factors affect the risk for superficial pressure ulcers: A mathematical modeling study. J Tissue Viability. 2018;27(1):27-35.

•Moore Z, Johanssen E, van Etten M, et al. Identifying the qualities of a pressure ulcer prevention care bundle: A systematic review. Int Wound J. 2020;17(3):800-812.
•Coyer F, Gardner A, Doubrovsky A, et al. Reducing pressure injuries in critically ill patients by using a patient skin integrity care bundle (InSPIRE): A quality improvement initiative. Intensive Crit Care Nurs. 2018;45:51-60.

•VanGilder C, Amlung S, Harrison P, et al. Results of the 2008-2009 International Pressure Ulcer Prevalence Survey and a 3-year, acute care, unit-specific analysis. Ostomy Wound Manage. 2009;55(11):39-45.

TABLE OF CONTENTS

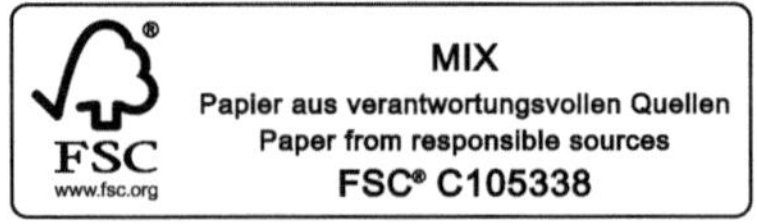

Printed by Books on Demand GmbH, Norderstedt / Germany